Kama Sutra Sex Positions

An Extensive Guide to Tantric and Kama Sutra Sex for Couples at All Levels (2022 Crash Course)

Zea Dean

Table of Contents

Kama Sutra Sex Positions

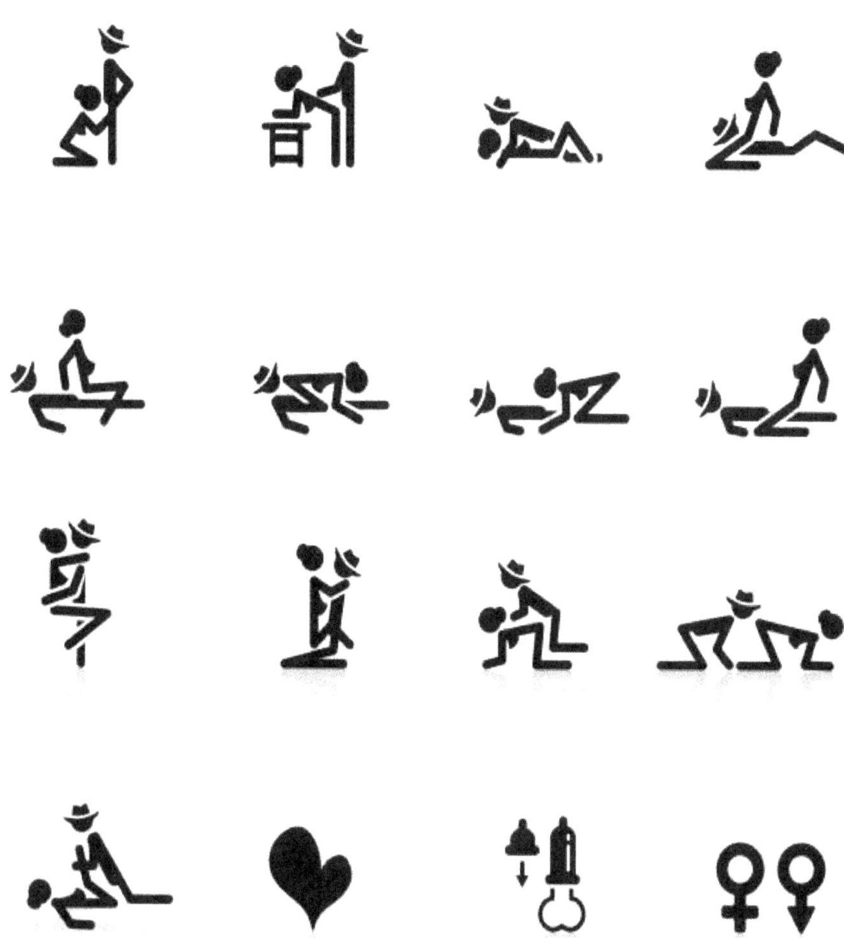

Chapter 1 Learning to Make Love

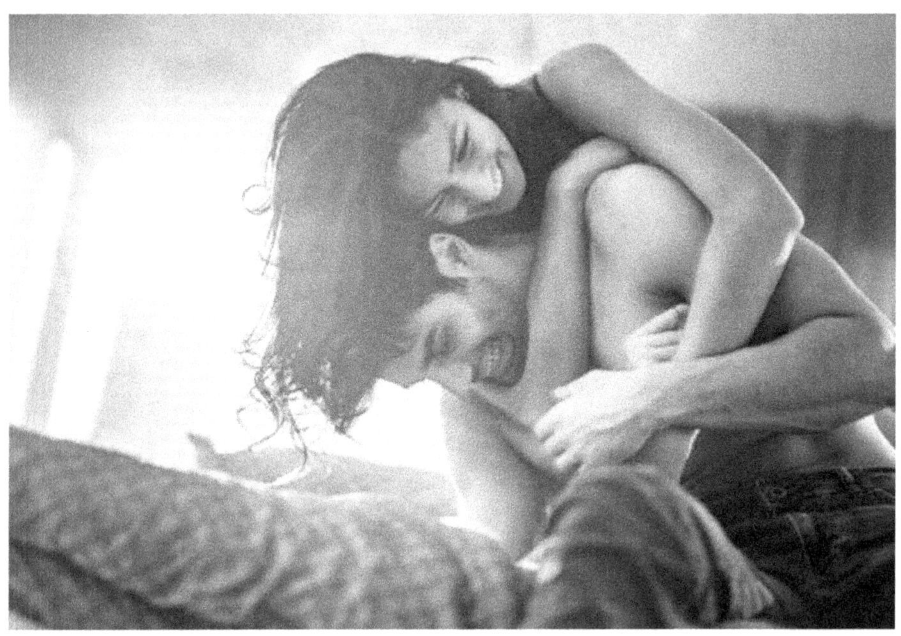

When you first start making love for the first time, you may feel uneasy, unsure of what positions to take or what the other person likes. You may feel pressure to outperform or satisfy your lover in ways they have never been satisfied before. All of these notions are reasonable, but it is uncommon for someone to become an expert the first time, or even the first ten times, they try anything new. The nice thing about sex is that it is a natural behavior for people to partake in, which means you will have some intrinsic understanding of how to behave oneself in a sexual experience. Keeping this in mind, you'll need to be able to trust yourself and your body to get the most out of your first few sexual encounters.

What You Should Know If This Is Your First Time

When it comes to your first sexual experience, there are a few things you should be aware of. Following on from the last point, the first thing to remember is to trust yourself! Humans are, at their most basic, animals. We are designed to have sex, just like every other animal. This indicates that sex is hardwired into our DNA and that we all have some idea of how to behave during sexual intercourse. This is due to our body's ability to take control and follow its pleasure, arousal, and impulses. While you don't want to behave like a full beast in bed (unless you and your partner are into it), this is just something to keep in mind to keep your anxieties in check. If you allow your mind to take control, it will obstruct and limit this natural inclination that you were born with.

This brings us to the next point to consider: relaxation and ease will make the experience much more pleasurable for both of you. If you can relax and enjoy the experience, your body will flow much more smoothly, and pleasure will come much more easily to both you and your partner.

The necessity of foreplay is the next point to mention. In case you're wondering, foreplay refers to any and all sexual acts that occur before the actual act of sexual intercourse. This may involve making out and groping, hand jobs or fingering, oral sex, or whatever else you do before penetration happens. This portion of sex is equally as crucial as the rest of it since it is when you get excited and allow your excitement to develop before starting to penetrate. This is the period when you may explore each other's body and discover where the other person likes to be touched the most. This aspect of sex is extremely significant for women, but we shall discuss it more in the next chapter.

The last point to mention for the first time is communication. It may seem that there is an expectation that you know precisely what you are doing and that you have done it a thousand times before, but this is not the case. No matter who your spouse is, they will appreciate that you spoke with them and made sure they were comfortable throughout the process rather than acting as if you knew precisely what they wanted. It's more amazing to be able to speak in bed than to be silent and guess the whole time.

Positions to Consider If This Is Your First Time

We'll now look at the greatest sex positions to try for the first time. With so many different sex positions to test, it might be difficult to determine which ones to try first. In this part, I'll discuss and detail the optimal positions to take during your first few sexual experiences. Remember that many individuals continue to have intercourse in these positions long after their first time, simply because they get the greatest pleasure from them. These aren't only for your first few sexual experiences, particularly if you like them so much.

Missionary

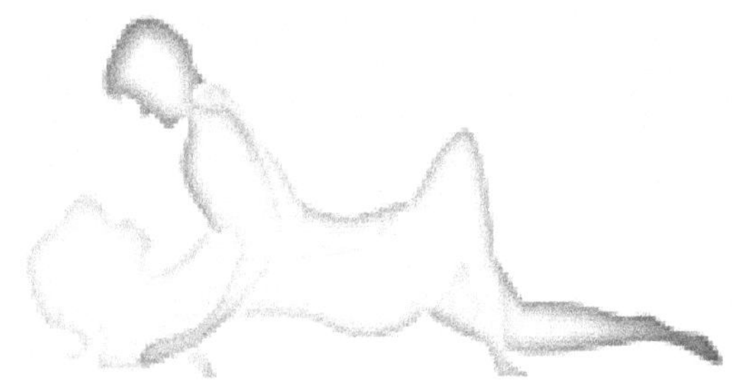

The Missionary position is one that you have most certainly heard about a thousand times. It is also known as the fundamental or starting posture. It has a horrible reputation for being the most boring of all positions. The missionary position, on the other hand, maybe really hot and passionate if you make it so! Here, I'll show you how to do this position and how it may provide you and your partner with hours of pleasure.

To begin, we will look at what the Missionary Position entails. When the lady rests on her back on the bed, she achieves this posture. The guy then lays on top of her, his face directly in front of hers. The male rests with his legs between the woman's and enters his penis from the front inside her. He controls the movement in and out with his hips while lying on top of the lady and holding his weight up with his arms. As I previously said, this posture may be intense if you want it to be. Because the man and woman are face-to-face, this is a very personal position. The closeness of your faces being so close together while you are in such a vulnerable posture leads to a strong connection and a lot of enjoyment. You may make out with your lover in this position to make it even more sensuous. If you're in a relationship while making love, you may stare deeply into each other's eyes, wink at them from time to time, or offer a little flirting grin.

When it feels amazing, tell your spouse by saying "oh yes" into their ear, breathing "oh yes" into their ear, or placing your lips near to their ear so they can hear your groaning up close. You may even nibble on their earlobes and lightly kiss their delicate neck skin, or you can go in for an intense kiss.

Missionary work may be as diverse and entertaining as you make it.

If you are confined to missionary work due to movement, flexibility, or other factors, you may utilize these strategies to keep it interesting for both you and your partner. If you are in a new relationship or having casual sex, you can penetrate in this position with your faces farther apart, perhaps kissing now and then, and as you become more comfortable with each other, you can gradually increase the level of intimacy and emotional connection by trying some of these ways of spicing it up and watch your relationship blossom.

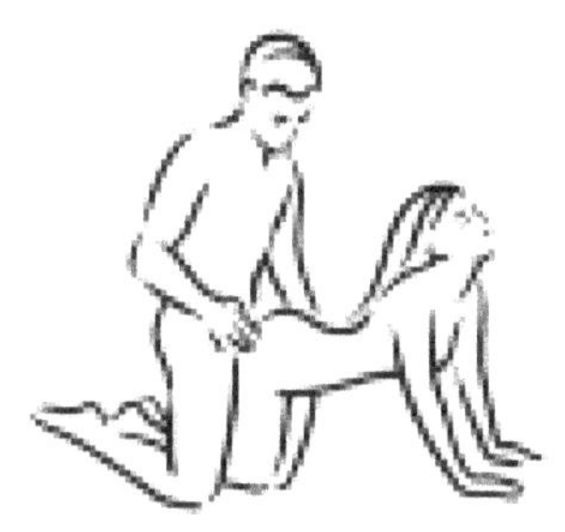

Doggy

The doggy style position is popular among both men and women. This posture may provide extreme pleasure to both men and women because the angles at which their genitals meet produce harmonious pleasure.

To get into this position, the lady goes down on her hands and knees on the bed (or sofa, or floor; this position works anyplace), and the guy gets down on his knees behind her, both facing the same way.

He will then approach her from behind. In this position, the male has control over the depth and pace of penetration. He may regulate the tempo by thrusting his hips. He grips her hips for a more powerful thrust and pulls her body closer to his if she wants him to go deeper.

Doggy fashion is a posture that ladies might like a lot. It's no wonder that it's a popular choice among young people of both genders. Because of the curvature of the man's erect penis and the angle at which it enters the woman's vagina, each thrust is extremely likely to activate her G-spot.

Because of the G-spot stimulation, the woman is extremely likely to have an orgasm as a result of the penetration. G spot stimulation may cause a woman to experience an extreme full-body pleasure for a long time before she has an orgasm. Hitting her G-spot will continue to feel fantastic for both the lady and the guy until one or both of them can no longer wait any longer and ultimate pleasure is attained. Keep in mind that we will go over the G-Spot in more detail in the next chapter.

Cowgirl

The Cowgirl position is the next one we'll look at. As you are surely aware, it is far more difficult for a woman to achieve orgasm via penetration than it is for a male. As a result, it is critical to understand which positions might maximize female enjoyment. If your female partner has difficulty achieving orgasm via penetrative sex alone, this position may lead to her feeling immense pleasure and attaining orgasm more readily than many other positions. The Cowgirl Position is similar to The Missionary Position in that both persons lie down with their faces only inches apart. Cowgirl, on the other hand, has the woman on top and is straddling the male.

To achieve this position, the guy will lay on his back on the bed, with the woman straddling his waist. From here, he may put his penis inside her. With the woman on top, she may control the angle of the man's penis within her by gliding and sliding her hips in the direction and motion that feels the most comfortable to her. She may keep moving in the direction and location that feels greatest to her to achieve orgasm.

Instead of reclining her upper body onto her partner, she may sit her body erect and move up and down on him in this posture if she prefers. As a result, you may make this position as personal or as public as you choose.

Cowgirl in Motion

This is a more sophisticated variation of the preceding classic posture, cowgirl. This position starts in the same manner as that. The male is on his back on the bed, and the lady is straddling his penis and pushing it inside her. The lady will move her hips on his penis to regulate the depth and pace of entry, allowing her to manage her enjoyment here. Because of the angle at which the man's penis touches the woman's vagina, this position is ideal for G-Spot stimulation. Because the penis bends upward and the G-Spot is located at the front of the vagina, postures with the man and woman's heads at the same end of the bed are ideal for G-Spot stimulation.

This position is advanced because, once in this position, you will introduce a vibrator to the woman's clitoris.

This may be done by either a guy or a woman, depending on your preference. Because the lady is sitting upright and on top, her clitoris is uncovered and therefore open and accessible to a vibrator. This will provide the lady with the most pleasure since she will get both G-Spot and clitoral stimulation at the same time.

She may even be able to reach a blended orgasm, which is the simultaneous occurrence of two separate orgasms, resulting in a massive mind-blowing climax. If you don't have a vibrator, you may stimulate the clitoris with your fingers (either the lady or the male).

Best Places for Intimacy

As previously said, closeness is something that must be worked on and developed. It is something that must be actively maintained and does not remain unchanged once accomplished.

There are numerous methods for a couple to improve their connection, and sex is one of them.

Sex has many additional advantages, but the positions we will look at today were picked because they are the greatest for generating closeness and connection between you and your partner.

Positions of the Kama Sutra for Anal Sex

The positions listed below are ideal for persons who are new to anal sex and want to attempt some of the basic positions to get acquainted with the sensation of anal sex. These postures are either directly from the Kama Sutra or are small adaptations of Kama Sutra positions that have been improved for anal sex.

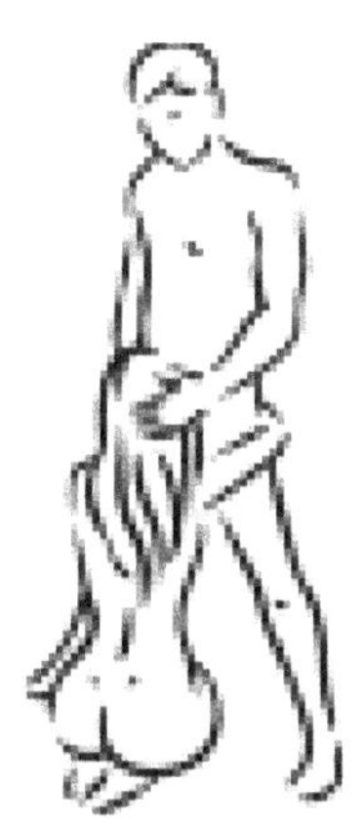

Oral Stimulation with Anal Stimulation

This initial position does not include anal penetration with a penis, but it is a terrific way to get started with anal play. When a woman performs oral sex on a guy, she assumes this posture. The guy rises, and the lady is on her knees in front of him, performing oral sex on him. She will then reach around behind the man's buttocks and use her finger to stimulate his anus. She may glide her finger over the outside of his anus, stimulating the delicate skin there and making him feel ecstatic. Giving him oral sex while also stroking his anus will make it almost difficult for him not to climax very fast.

Angel with Curled Hair

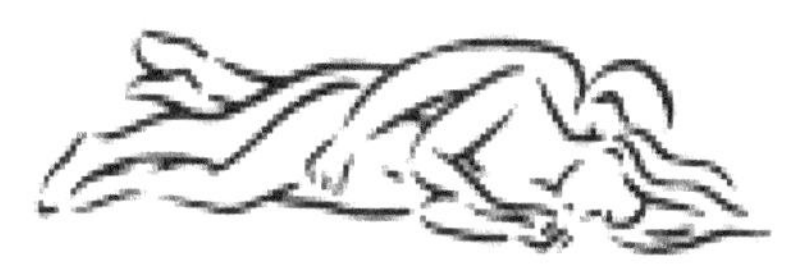

This is a Kama Sutra position that is intended to be performed with vaginal intercourse, but it may also be performed with anal sex. The man and lady are laying down on their sides, with the man behind the woman.

Because they are both facing the same direction, the curvature of their hips positions the man's penis at the ideal spot for anal entry. In this position, the man and woman may press their hips into each other, and control is a joint effort.

The Clip

The guy is lying back on the bed with his knees bent and his feet placed on the bed in this posture. The lady sits on top of the guy and pushes his penis into her anus. In this position, the woman may lean forward for support and control the depth and pace of penetration by leaning forward onto the man's bowed legs. The male may grip the woman's buttocks and direct her motions.

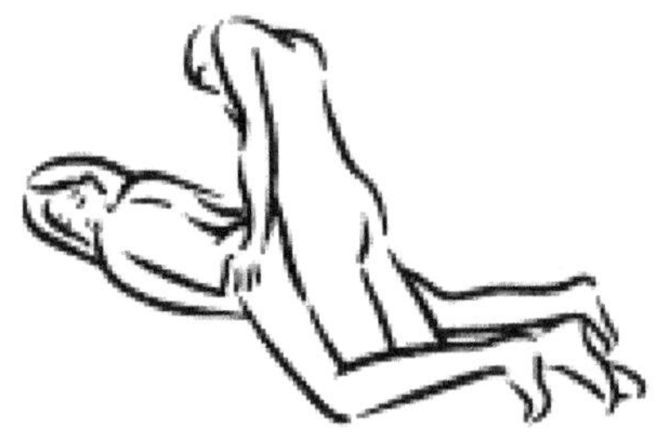

The snake

When you have some experience with anal sex but aren't ready to attempt anything too intense, this is a decent position to try. In this position, the individual receiving anal penetration plays a passive role and may concentrate on relaxing and enjoying the pleasure rather than needing to contort into some sort of acrobatic shape.

To begin, the lady will lay face down on the bed, and her boyfriend will lie on top of her, his arms supporting him. From here, the lady will arch her back slightly to make her pleasure zones as accessible to penetration as feasible. The male will now carefully insert his penis into her anus. Without having to do anything, the lady may enjoy the pleasure journey her lover takes her on. She can relish these times when all attention is on her!

Pegging

There is another sort of anal sex available, which utilizes sex toys. It is not uncommon for a woman to anally enter her male partner while wearing a strap-on. This is referred to as Pegging. You're ready to attempt Pegging now that you've learned a bit more about sex toys and anal sex, as well as how to combine the two safely and hygienically. This may be accomplished by inserting a dildo inside a woman's strap-on or by utilizing a double-ended dildo. Using a double-ended dildo allows the woman to be pleasured while entering the guy since she will be entered vaginally or anally with the other end of the dildo. This dildo appears like any other, except for the fact that it has two identical ends.

You can comprehend how any of these anal sex positions may be accomplished by either the man piercing the woman anally with his penis or the woman penetrating her partner anally with a dildo now that you are aware of the feasibility of this sort of practice.

Anal intercourse is highly enjoyable for males because anal penetration stimulates their prostate. The prostate is referred regarded as the "male G-Spot."

Chapter 2: Effective Kama Sutra Sex Positions for Male Orgasm

The postures in this chapter have been selected for their advantages to male orgasm in particular.

The Closed Door

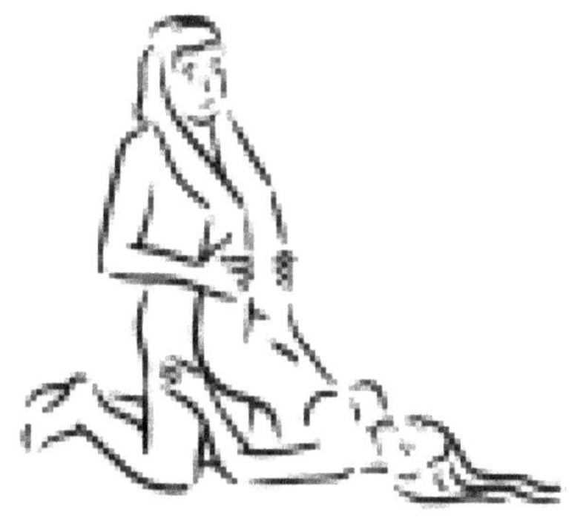

This position is similar to the missionary in that both persons are laying face to face, with the male on top. The distinction, and what distinguishes this as an advanced position, is that the lady will maintain her legs closed firmly the whole time.

The man's penis may be entered while her legs are open, and she will shut her legs after it is in. This constricts her vagina and tightens the canal for the man's penis. Furthermore, if she is excited, her vagina will get engorged and the canal will become much tighter. As a result, the man's penis will be held intimately as it slips in and out of her, providing added pleasure for him.

Lap Dancing

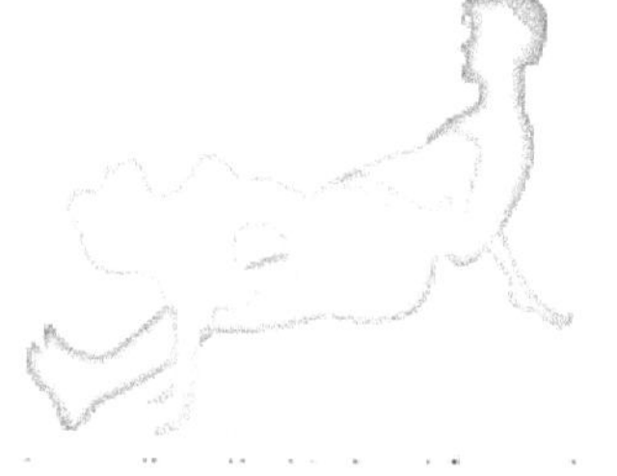

This is another posture that is ideal for male pleasure and male orgasm. This position involves strength from both the man and the woman and is highly athletic, which is why it is referred to be an advanced sex position. When attempting this, use caution.

To get into position, the male will sit erect in a comfortable chair or on the edge of a bed, his feet on the floor.

The lady will get upon his lap and either wrap her legs behind him or push her legs straight out beyond him. The guy may then put his penis into the woman's vaginal opening. From here, the lady will recline back until her body is flat and she is laying straight back.

Depending on your height variances, the male will have to hold onto her at her hips or lower back as she performs this. The male in this posture will press his hips into the lady from a sitting position while repeatedly dragging her onto his penis. A great level of upper body strength is needed of the guy in this position. When attempting this position, place some cushions on the floor underneath the lady just in case.

In this case, the lady may also lean on the man's arms for support.

This position is excellent for the male's enjoyment since it enables him to regulate the pace and depth of his thrusting, as well as deep penetration, which will feel fantastic on his penis.

Dividing the Bamboo

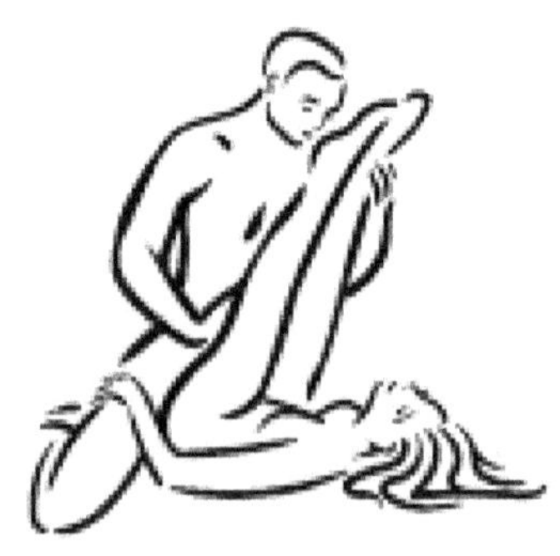

This is the basic Kama Sutra position, and it is ideal for male orgasms. To achieve this posture, the lady will lay on her back on the bed and extend one of her legs straight out under her, raising the other leg and putting it on the man's shoulder. The male will be laying on top of the lady, his hips wedged between her legs.

Because of the location of the woman's legs, the guy can achieve deep penetration in this position, which will feel fantastic for him. The deeper he can go, the more satisfied he will be.

If the lady is not flexible enough to do this posture in this manner, the guy might kneel instead of resting on top of her.

The posture is still achieved in this manner, but the woman's leg is not stretched as much. This posture is especially advantageous for women since the likelihood of G-Spot activation is quite high.

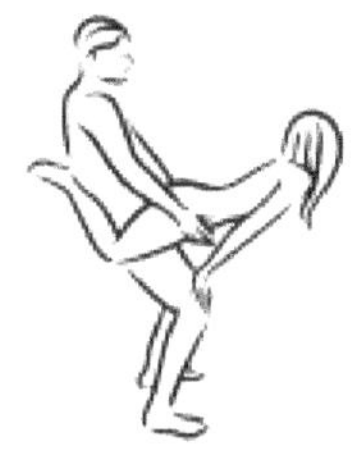

Anal-Standing Suspended from Behind

This position is ideal for anal sex veterans since it allows for deep penetration while also requiring strength from both parties. This one is a little difficult to get into, so start by having the guy sit on the edge of the bed or in a chair, and the lady sits on his lap, facing away from him. The male will next push his penis into her anus. He'll grab her beneath her legs or under her buttocks, and once she's secure, he'll rise, still within her.

Then, while resting against a wall for support, he would push into and out of her, holding her up. If fitness and strength are present, this position may be quite delightful for both persons, which is why it is such an advanced position. This position is ideal for male orgasms since the position, as well as the fact that it includes anal intercourse, will make him feel fantastic. The only problem is that it takes a significant amount of effort on the part of the lady.

Chapter 3 Kama Sutra Sex Positions for Female Orgasm

The postures that follow are ideal for female orgasm and female pleasure. Positions that enhance G-Spot contact and allow for simultaneous clitoral stimulation provide the most enjoyment for the woman.

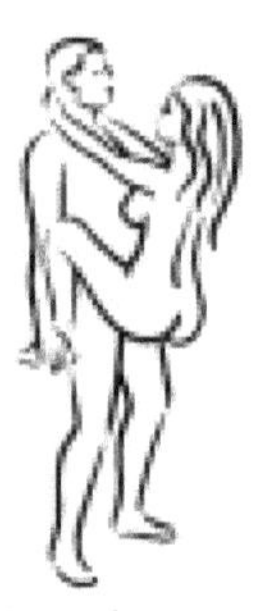

Suspended Standing

This initial position is derived from the Kama Sutra. This position is ideal for female orgasm due to the angle at which the man's penis enters her vagina, as well as the fact that the guy is in charge in this position, allowing the woman to relax and enjoy the pleasure he is delivering to her body.

To get into this position, the guy will face a wall while the lady stands in front of him with her back to the wall. She will then leap into his arms, wrapping both her arms and legs around him.

He may then put his penis into her vagina while holding onto her buttocks or beneath her knees. He may rest her back against the wall in front of him for support, avoiding having to hold her full weight in his arms. Holding onto her under her knees will open her up and provide easy access to her vagina.

The fact that she is suspended, along with this, will result in deep penetration, which will be delightful for both the man and the lady. Deep penetration is excellent for female orgasm because there are two locations deep inside the vagina that, when stimulated, result in a highly strong orgasm for a woman.

In order for this to happen, the penis must maintain continuous deep penetration, which is entirely doable in this posture.

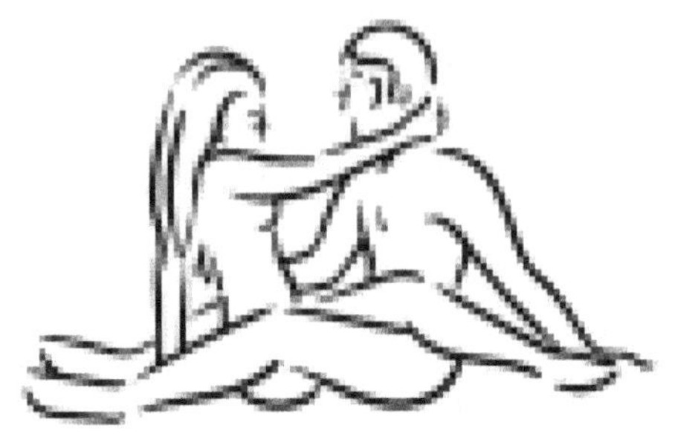

Vibrating Cross-Legged

Because it incorporates both penetration and clitoral stimulation, this position allows for several female orgasms. The male will sit cross-legged, while the lady will sit on his lap, her legs wrapped around behind him. This may be done in a relaxing chair or on a bed.

Once the penis is within the woman's vagina, he may shove into her with his hips or use his arms to raise her up and down on his penis.

She may then use a vibrator on her clitoris (or her hand if she doesn't have one) since her legs are spread wide in a cross-legged stance. This posture allows for G-Spot stimulation as well as clitoral stimulation, which may result in a blended orgasm. It may also result in several orgasms. This may happen if she comes clitorally and then continues to penetrate, which might lead to a G-Spot orgasm (or general vaginal orgasm). Then there's the chance she'll have another clitoral orgasm if she starts stroking her clitoris again.

Scissors

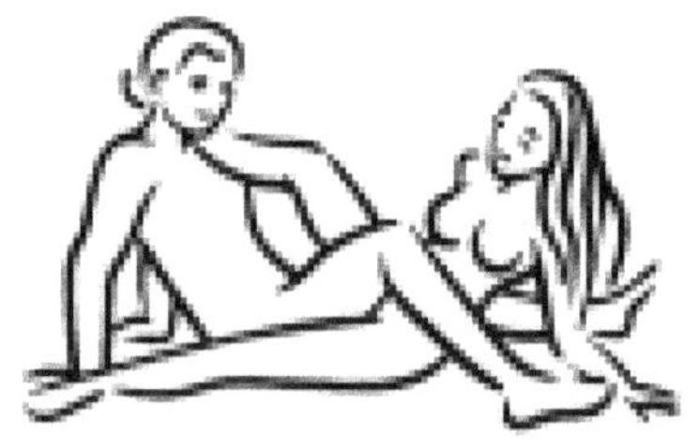

This is a challenging position to get, but once obtained, it will be well worth the effort. To begin, the male will sit on the bed, arms behind his back, keeping his weight up but leaning back. Then he will bend one of his knees, bending his leg.

The lady will lay face down on the bed, her head at the opposite end of the bed as the men. She'll widen her legs and bring her body closer to the man's till their bodies collide. When they collide, their bodies will resemble two pairs of scissors crossed. The male will next push his penis inside her vagina. The lady is able to move her body up and down on his penis, while the male is able to push into her. It may take some time to establish a rhythm in this position, but once you do, you will both experience an immense pleasure.

This takes us to the next type of position, which is the finest for several female orgasms.

Chapter 4 Kama Sutra: Tantric Positions for Her Pleasure

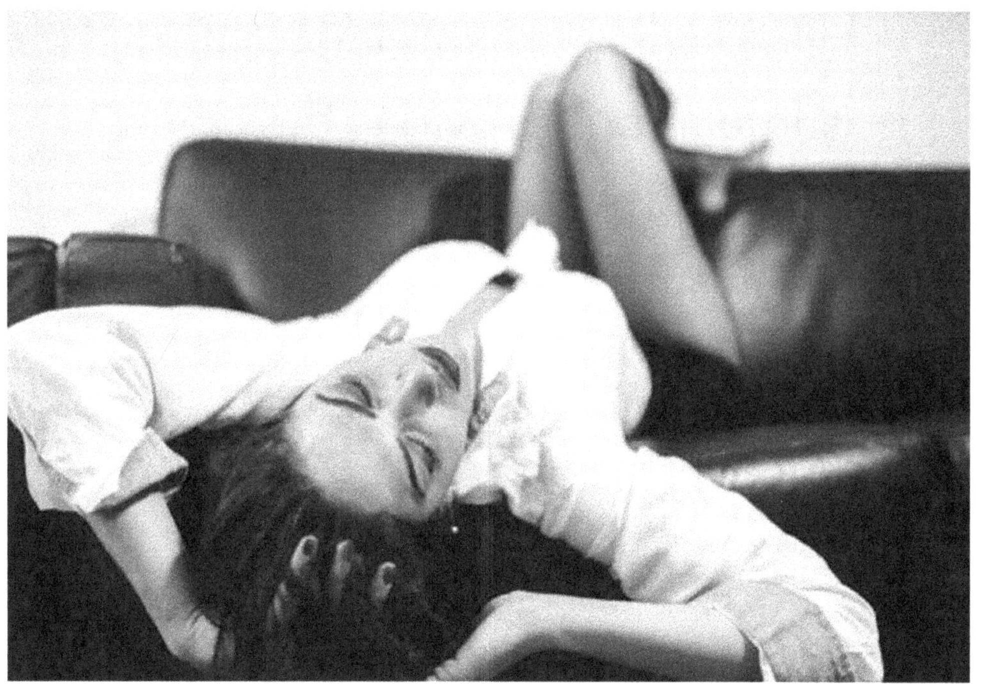

The postures that follow are ideal for female orgasm and female pleasure. Positions that enhance G-Spot contact and allow for simultaneous clitoral stimulation provide the most enjoyment for the woman.

The Peasant

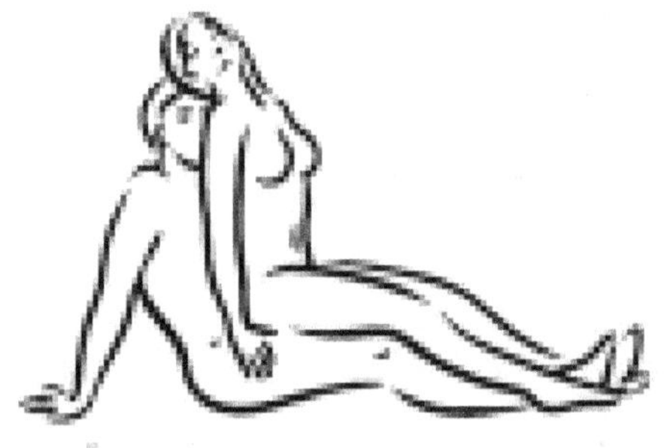

This position is ideal for a woman because it provides both clitoral stimulation and penetration. To achieve this posture, the guy will sit on the floor or bed, while the lady will sit on top of his lap.

The lady will spread her legs wide, and the male will enter his penis from behind inside her. While the lady grinds on his lap, the male will reach around her and rub her clitoris.

The Position of the Rider

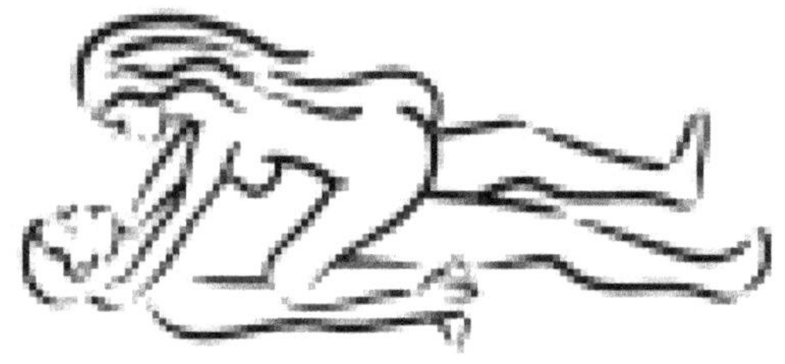

The male will lay on his back and stretch his legs wide to his chest. The lady will next sit on the man's penis, below his bowed legs. She may balance herself on his bent legs, grind on his penis, or raise her body up and down on him. This posture is ideal for female enjoyment since she may touch or have the guy stimulate her clitoris. It's also enjoyable for her since she has control over the movement.

Indrani

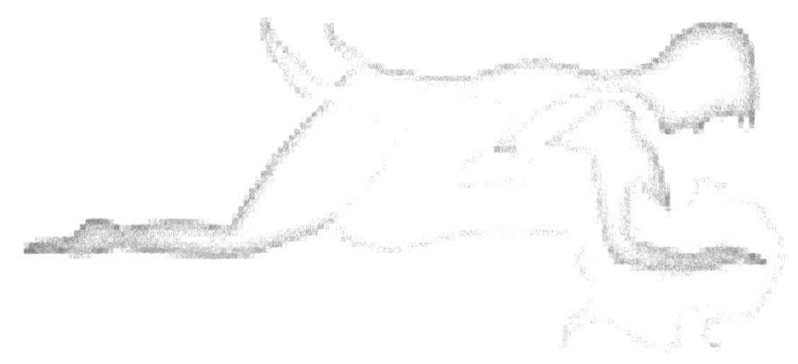

This is a more acrobatic posture than many other Kama Sutra poses. The lady will lay on her back, with the male kneeling in front of her, near her legs. The male will grab her buttocks and insert his penis inside her. He'll grab her thighs to keep her buttocks up off the bed. This posture causes disruptions and shifts in blood flow, giving the lady a great deal of pleasure.

The Position of Yawning

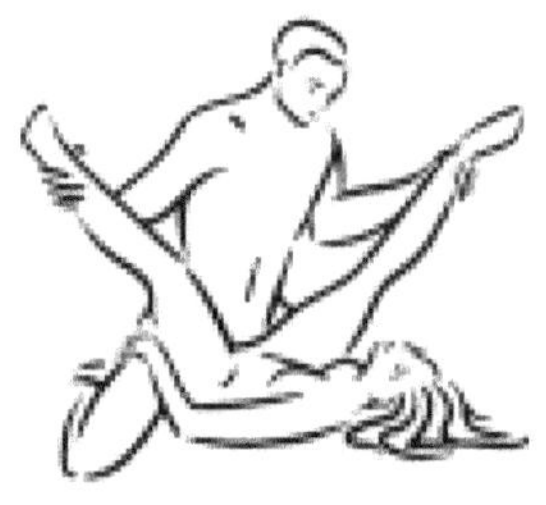

The lady lays on her back, spreading her legs as much as she can. The male will approach the lady from the front, his knees under her hips. In this posture, he may bend forward and their faces can come close together.

The Strolling Horse

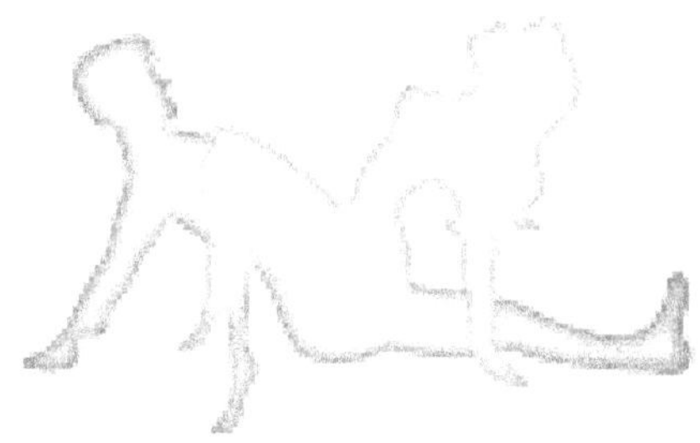

This is a female-dominated job. Because the angle of the man's penis inside of her will contact her G-Spot, she will be able to experience pleasure more easily. The guy sits on the floor, arms extending behind him. The lady will sit on the man's back, facing him. To control the thrusting, she would grasp his thighs with hers and manipulate her hips. Because they are both sitting up, this posture allows for a close hug.

The Crucifixion

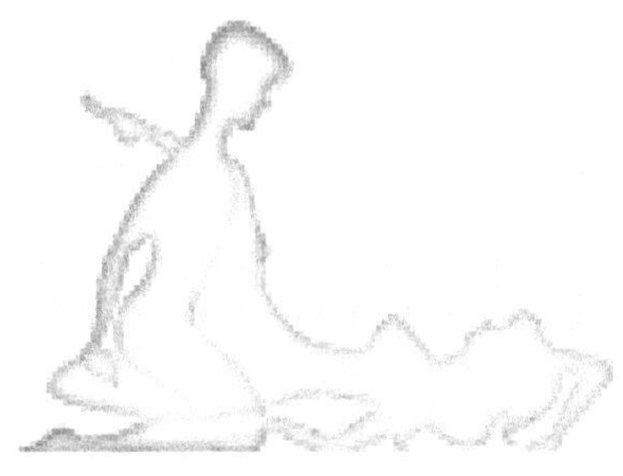

The lady is lying on her back, one leg straight up in the air. The guy kneels in front of her, straddling her stretched leg on the bed and holding onto her other leg in the air.

He may then advance his body between her two legs till he is near enough to implant his penis inside her vagina. He may spread her legs with his body, straddling one and resting the other on his shoulder. His hands will be free to play with her clitoris, touch her breasts, running his hands up and down her body, or do anything they like.

Chapter 5 The Kama Sutra Tantric Positions for His Pleasure

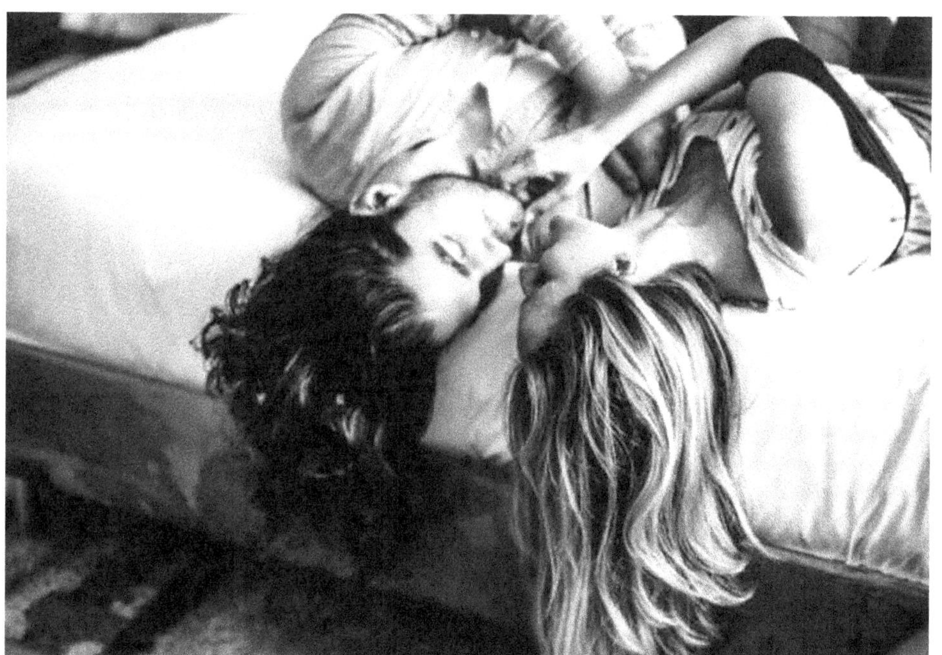

Position of the Mare

This is a posture derived from The Kama Sutra. More than the position itself, this position is excellent for a man's enjoyment because of the skill involved on the side of the lady. This approach has the ability to completely transform your sexual life.

The guy sits in this posture with his legs out in front of him and his arms back, resting his weight on the bed. The lady straddles him and lays herself onto his hard penis, facing him. Once the man's penis is within her, the woman utilizes her vaginal muscles to exert and relieve pressure on the man's penis, almost as if she's milking it. This is where the name came from. Because it exerts changing pressure when he is piercing her, this method produces incredibly delightful feelings on the man's penis. It stimulates the man's penis more than traditional penetration. As an added benefit, this strengthens the woman's vaginal muscles, which will lead to bigger orgasms for her in the future.

Position of the Tripod

This is a standing posture for both the lady and the male.

The lady and guy will face one other, and the male will grab one of the woman's legs beneath her knee. The male will elevate her leg and enter her from below. The Tripod Position is so named because there are just three legs on the ground. This posture promotes maximal blood flow to the genitals, resulting in intense male enjoyment.

Position of Piditaka

This is another Kama Sutra posture that needs some flexibility but is really calming once you've mastered it. The lady reclines on the bed and places her knees on the man's chest. The male will climb on top of the lady, pressing her knees towards his chest. The male will enter her from this posture, with his knees on each side of her buttocks. This position is ideal for male enjoyment since the vagina is restricted and the woman's legs are raised, which feels amazing on his penis.

Position of hanging

This posture is comparable to standing, however, it differs in that it requires a bit more support. The male will stand with his back to a wall, and the lady will stand facing him. The lady will leap into the man's arms, and he will support her on her buttocks. The lady will stretch her legs behind her and rest them on the wall. The guy enjoys this position because the woman's vagina is closed, creating a tighter environment for the penis.

The Slanted Position

The lady will lay on the floor and raise her legs, bringing her knees to her chest and spreading them. She will grip her legs under her knees to keep them raised. To enter the lady from below, the guy will kneel down in a squat stance and lean forward. As he thrusts inside her, he may grip onto her legs for support. This posture feels amazing on the man's penis since the woman's legs are elevated.

The Cow Posture

The Cow Position is one in which the guy enters the lady from behind. The lady will lay face down on a bed with a cushion under her hips to elevate her buttocks slightly off the bed. The male will climb over the lady and penetrate her. This position is excellent for male enjoyment since it allows him to regulate speed and depth.

Putting A Nail Back Together

The lady will lay on her back, and the male will climb over her and raise one of her legs. He will raise her leg so that her foot rests on his brow. He may then enter her from the front while her foot is on his head. As he thrusts into her, she will alternate her feet on his head, changing the emotions for both of them and offering variety.

The Pinch

The guy is on his side, and the lady is on her side, facing him, with her head toward his feet. The lady will raise her knees to her chest and lay one of her legs underneath and the other on top of the man's legs. She is essentially embracing his legs with her whole body. She glides up till her vulva is very near to his penis. When he is correctly oriented, he can penetrate her and attain depth and control since she is precisely positioned for his penis to enter her. The lady wraps her arms around his legs, allowing him to use his hands and arms to assist with thrusting.

Chapter 6 The Menstrual Cycle and Sex

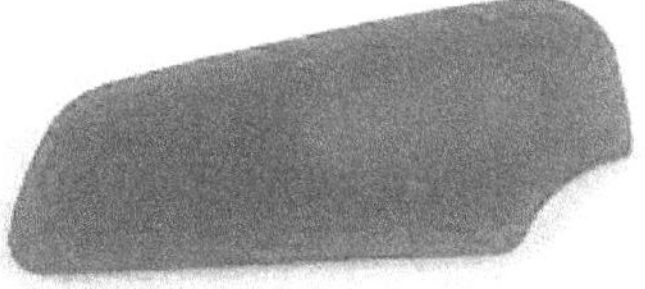

Menstrual Cycle Basics

Every month, a lady gets her period while she is younger. Period is the colloquial name for menstruation, and it will be used afterwards. If a woman does not get pregnant, she will have her period once a month, during which the lining of her uterus will be shed. This opens the door to the potential of pregnancy the next month, since the uterus will produce new cells throughout the month. A period normally lasts around a week and includes the discharge of skin cells and blood via the vagina. This is because extra skin and blood gather in the uterus to prepare for a prospective pregnancy, but it only lasts for one month at a time.

The Advantages and How It Affects Sex

If a lady feels at ease, having sex during her period is not an issue. There is nothing that says a woman cannot, and it will not harm either the male or the woman. The only difference, as long as neither of them is terrified of blood, will be the mess that it will create. Women really have a substantially stronger sex urge during their cycles and the week before them.

There are certain advantages to having sex during your period. One of these advantages is that having sex while on your period might help relieve the agony of period cramps. Period cramps may be very painful, and anything that helps them feel better, particularly when it feels as wonderful as sex, is a welcome proposal. This is the outcome of the orgasm. The chemicals generated in the brain make you joyful and also have pain-relieving properties. The uterus contracts and then releases as a result of an orgasm. In terms of cramping, the releasing portion of this will most likely make a lady feel better than she did before.

Another advantage of having an orgasm during your period is that it causes the uterus to contract, which forces the blood and uterine contents out quicker, resulting in a shorter period duration. This also implies that there is sufficient natural lubrication and that lubricant is not required during period sex.

Best Kama Sutra Positions to Experiment with During Menstruation

Showering is a fantastic place to have sex during menstruation. This reduces the amount of cleaning required, and any blood that gets on either of you may be rinsed off straight immediately. This is a cleaner and more pleasant option than having sex in bed and then having to hop in the shower.

Shower sex is also steamy (literally) and hot (literally), which may make for some really enjoyable body-on-body activity. Make sure the water is at the proper temperature and that you have a mat or something on the floor to prevent sliding! Before you begin any form of water penetration, make sure you use enough of waterproof lube since the water in the shower will not be enough of a lubricant for the interior of a vagina and will actually produce unpleasant friction. Let's prevent that from happening; lubricant is your buddy!

Doggy Style Standing

Standing Doggy Style is a variation on the Kama Sutra pose. It's a nice place to start with shower sex since it keeps you from being blasted in the face with a hot stream of water while you're trying to concentrate on having a happy orgasm.

Doggy Style in the Shower is a unique twist on an old classic that is enjoyable for both parties.

The guy stands with his back to the rushing water, facing away from the lady who stands in front of him. The lady then leans forward, her hands on the side of the tub or the shower wall for support. The guy pushes his penis inside her from behind, holding her hips for a deeper thrust, and they're ready to proceed. This position provides a considerable likelihood of the male being able to hit the woman's G-spot with his penis, thus the lady will appreciate it a lot. The warmth and moist atmosphere of the shower will undoubtedly result in a wonderful sexual session.

Shower Sex Position Kama Sutra

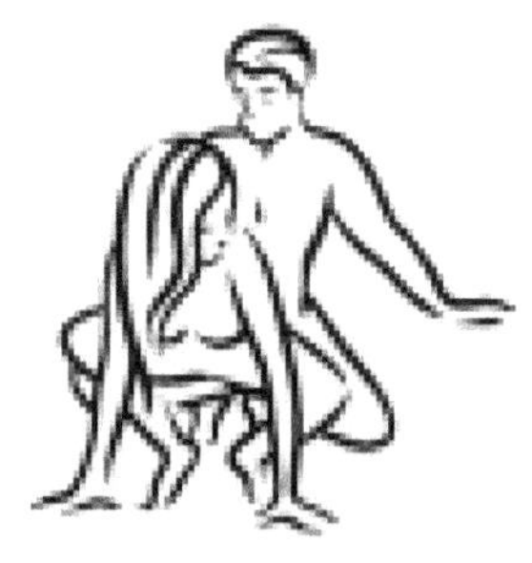

This is another position to experiment with in the shower. If you and your partner are looking for a position that doesn't need you to concentrate too much on challenging posture and keeping yourself up in a slippery shower, you might attempt the kneeling position. Have you both kneeled on the shower floor, one behind the other? You may travel in a variety of directions from here. You may utilize this posture as foreplay by reaching around with your hands to enjoy each other's genitals before moving to the bedroom together. You can also use this as foreplay before moving to another position in the shower for penetration. You may also begin penetrating straight away. You'll need to adjust your knee heights to line up your erection and her vagina beautifully for effortless penetration. This position is full of options and is a really hot way to get you both in the mood for whatever comes next, whether in or out of the shower.

Chair that bounces

This is not a shower position, but it is ideal for sex during her period. This is due to the fact that it may be done on the floor, making cleanup easier.

To achieve this posture, the male will sit on the floor (on towels or sheets to make cleaning easier) and sit back on his heels. The lady will sit on his lap, facing him, and he will insert his penis inside her. She'll keep her feet on the ground and use them to bounce herself up and down on the man's penis. This position is ideal because the woman is hovering over the floor, allowing the majority of the blood to land there rather than all over the bed or the man.

Things to Remember
There are a few things to consider if you and your partner decide to have sex during your period.

1. Bloodstaining

If you are going to have sex someplace other than the bathtub or shower, be sure you lay down a lot of towels or anything that can absorb the blood before you begin. It will stain your white bed linens if you get it on them. Maintain in mind that whichever towels you choose to set down will almost certainly get discolored, so choose ones that you don't need to keep freshly white.

2. Self-Awareness

Having sex during a woman's menstruation might make her feel self-conscious. Keeping this in mind is critical since she may be sensitive to her body or the quantity of blood involved.

3. Infections Spreaded Through Sexual Contact

It is vital to understand that certain STIs are spread via the blood. These are either HIV or hepatitis. To be safe, it is essential to wear condoms at all times, but particularly when there will be blood involved during sex.

Fur tampons

Tampons that are left at home when having sex can be problematic. If you were using a tampon before having intercourse, make sure you remove it before inserting a penis or fingers into the vagina. Otherwise, a doctor will be required to remove the tampon.

5. It's Still Possible to Get Pregnant

While the chances of becoming pregnant during your period are lower, you can still become pregnant during your period. It is impossible to predict when your body will be ready to conceive during your period, therefore proper safeguards are required.

www.ingramcontent.com/pod-product-compliance
Lightning Source LLC
LaVergne TN
LVHW020924200726
843506LV00011B/1798